25 PALEO LUNCHBOX RECIPES
ON-THE-GO RECIPES FOR A BUSY LIFESTYLE

Contents

About the Book

Today's world is a busy place and eating on the go isn't always that easy, especially for those who follow the guidelines of a Paleolithic diet. This book will help anyone on the Paleo diet, who wants to take their lunch to work or has children's lunchbox's to prepare. In the next section, there's an introduction explaining the basics of the Paleo diet and the benefits it provides. This is followed by a collection of 25 recipes to make it easy to be on the go and Paleo.

Introduction

Before the advent of agriculture and processed foods, our ancestors ate what they could hunt or forage for. This Paleolithic diet, also known as the cavemen diet, uses strict guidelines to provide the vitamins and minerals we need. It includes eating only organic meat, seafood, fruits, vegetables and nuts. It does not include grains, legumes or processed, sugary foods of any kind. Followers of the Paleo diet divide their daily intake into two sources, eating 40% from plants and 60% from animals.

The Paleo diet has exhibited many benefits to its followers, including reducing blood sugar problems, cardio vascular disease, intestinal problems and metabolic imbalances. As with any diet, it's important to feel satisfied after every meal and the Paleo diet is no exception. If your life is busy and you or family need to pack lunches each day, these recipes provide the healthy alternative you've been searching for, fill you up and taste great. Enjoy!

Sandwiches

Asian Chicken Wrap

4 servings

2 boneless chicken breasts, cooked and chopped

2 tbsp. organic, gluten-free soy sauce

1/4 small cabbage

4 carrots

1/4 pound snow peas

1 small Vidalia onion

1/4 c. finely chopped cilantro

1 small Vidalia onion, diced

1/3 c. sliced water chestnuts

8 large spinach leaves

In a medium bowl, mix together chopped chicken and soy sauce and set aside to marinate, while preparing the other ingredients. Chop the cabbage into thin ribbons. Slice carrots into thin matchsticks. Slice snow peas lengthwise. Dice onion. In a large bowl combine vegetables. Add water chestnuts and mix thoroughly. Pour chicken and soy sauce and toss to coat. Lay out a spinach leaf. Place a couple of spoonful's of the mixture in the center of the leaf. Fold bottom and top of leaf in over mixture. Fold one side of leaf and roll up like a burrito. Repeat for the other leaves

Bacon & Egg Salad Spread

4 servings

4 slices crisp-fried bacon, crumbled

5 large eggs, hardboiled and chopped

½ c. Paleo Mayo (see recipe below)

¼ c. onions

¼ c. celery

2 tsp. chopped green pepper

½ tsp. sea salt

¼ tsp. freshly ground pepper

Dash of paprika

Paleo Mayo:

Yolk of 1 large egg

¼ tsp. salt

¼ tsp. Dijon mustard

1 ½ tsp. lemon juice

1 tsp. apple cider vinegar

¾ c. extra virgin olive oil

In medium bowl, whisk together egg yolk, salt, mustard, lemon juice and vinegar. Once mixed thoroughly, add very slowly (drop by drop) the olive oil while continuing to whisk. Whisk mixture until all the oil is incorporated and the mixture turns into a white, creamy Paleo Mayo. (This can also be done in a food processor.)

Place all ingredients in a large bowl and mix thoroughly. Chill for 30 minutes. Spread on Paleo White Bread from recipe on page 9 or place a scoop on a lettuce leaf sprinkled with paprika and roll for a wrap.

Chicken Salad

4 servings

1 c. diced cooked chicken

¼ c. Paleo Mayo (from recipe on page 6)

¼ c. chopped onion

¼ c. chopped red bell pepper

½ c. diced pineapple

¼ chopped walnuts

Salt & pepper to taste

Mix all ingredients in a large bowl, Chill for up to an hour before serving.

Ham & Turkey Roll-Ups

1 Serving

2 Slices Ham

2 Slices Turkey

1 Olive

Toothpicks

Lay out one slice of ham. Place on top, one slice of turkey. Place on turkey the second slice of ham. Finish layering with the second slice of turkey. Roll up the slices. Spear an olive on a toothpick and secure ham/turkey roll up with toothpick. Keep closed with a toothpick. Make as many or as few as you want.

London Broil

4 Servings

2 c. almond meal

1/3 c. tapioca flour

1/2 c. chestnut flour

3/4 tsp. baking soda

1/4 tsp. salt

1/3 c. coconut oil

7 eggs, divided

1/3 c. coconut milk

2 tbsp. slightly warmed honey

London broil

1 London broil cut of beef

1/4 c. olive oil

Lettuce, Onion, Tomato Slices

To make bread: Preheat oven to 325°F. Grease the bottom and sides of an 8.5″ x 4.5″ bread loaf pan and line the bottom with parchment. Grease the parchment. Combine the flours, with the salt and baking soda. Pulse to combine. Add in the coconut oil, yolks and milk and pulse until smooth. Add the honey. In another bowl, beat the egg whites until firm but still wet. Blend about 1/3 of the egg white mixture into the almond mixture to lighten it somewhat (it will still be a thick paste). Fold in the remainder of the egg whites and almond mixture into one another. Transfer to the prepared pan. Bake for 40-45 minutes, or until set. Cool on rack. Slice for sandwiches.

Cut London broil into 2-inch slices, across the grain. Then butterfly the slices. In a large skillet, heat oil. Place meat in oil and brown on each side, cook until desired doneness.

Place meat between two slices of bread, adding lettuce, onions, and tomato as desired.

Roast Beef Roll Up

Serves 1

1 large Romaine lettuce leaf

1 tsp. pure mustard

1 thick slice cooked roast beef or 2 thin slices

1 slice avocado

1 slice tomato

Lay out lettuce leaf. Spread mustard on leaf. Place roast beef, lengthwise on leaf. Add avocado and tomato on top of meat. Roll up lengthwise.

Tuna Salad

4 Servings

1 5-oz. can tuna, packed in water

¼ c. Paleo Mayo (from page 6)

2 large eggs, hardboiled & diced

2 tbsp. chopped onion

2 tbsp. chopped celery

Drain tuna and set aside in medium bowl. Add a dollop of the mayonnaise to the tuna and mix well. Add in hardboiled eggs, onion and celery. Stir until well mixed, putting in more mayonnaise, if desired. Spread tuna salad on bread, using Paleo White Bread recipe on page 9 or place a scoop on a lettuce leaf, roll for a wrap.

Turkey Bacon Roll Up

1 serving

1 tbsp. apple cider vinegar

1 tbsp. + 1 tsp. mustard powder

¼ tsp. crushed mustard seeds

2 slices of roast turkey

2 slices crisp fried bacon

2 tsp. red onion, diced

2 tsp. tomato, diced

In a small bowl, mix vinegar, mustard powder and seeds together to form mustard. Spread mustard on one slices of turkey. Add slice of bacon, and 1 tsp. each of onion and tomato to edge of turkey slice and roll up. Make another for two rolls per serving.

Sides

Ants on a Log

1 serving

2 stalks celery

4 tbsp. almond butter

½ c. raisins

Wash and trim celery. Cut celery into halves or thirds. Spread almond butter in each section and sprinkle with raisins.

Beet Chips

4 servings

4 beets thinly sliced

¼ c. olive oil

Place sliced beets on backing sheet. Brush with olive oil. Bake at 350 degrees Fahrenheit for 20 minutes, turning about halfway through.

Carrot Apple Mint Salad

4 servings

3 tbsp. extra virgin olive oil, or oil of your choice

1 tbsp. wine vinegar

Sea salt & pepper to taste

¾ lb. carrots

½ lb. cabbage

3 sweet apples

2 heaping tbsp. fresh chopped chives

2 heaping tbsp. fresh chopped mint

Mix oil, vinegar, salt and pepper. Grate carrots, cabbage, and apples. (Easiest to grate in a food processor) In a large bowl, mix grated ingredients with chives and mint. Refrigerate before serving.

Coleslaw

6 servings

Dressing:

1/4 c. of honey

1/4 c. of apple cider vinegar

1/8 c. of balsamic vinegar

1 clove of garlic, finely minced

3 tbsp. olive oil

1/2 tsp. Dijon mustard

1/4 tsp. sea salt

1/4 tsp. black pepper

Coleslaw:

1/2 head of red cabbage, shredded

1 medium carrot, grated

1/2 green bell pepper, diced

In a small saucepan, combine the dressing ingredients and heat on medium-high heat, bringing the mixture to a boil, reduce heat to low and simmer for three minutes. Combine all the coleslaw ingredients and pour dressing over to evenly coat. Refrigerate for one hour before serving.

Cucumber Watermelon Salad

4 servings

1 tbsp. olive extra virgin olive oil

2 tsp. fresh lemon juice

¼ tsp. sea salt

1 c. thinly sliced cucumber

¼ c. vertically sliced onion

2 c. cubed watermelon

1 tbsp. fresh basil

Combine oil, lemon juice, and salt in large bowl. Stir well. Add watermelon, cucumber, and onion. Toss to coat. Sprinkle evenly with basil.

Fruit Cup

1 serving

1 orange, peeled and divided

1 tbsp. crushed pineapple

1 tbsp. diced pears

2 ripe cherries chopped

1 tbsp. shredded coconut

Mix all ingredients. Refrigerate until chilled and serve.

Radish Chips

4 servings

2 bunches radishes

¼ c. olive oil

Wash and trim radishes. Slice thin. Place in a single layer on a baking sheet. Brush radishes with olive oil. Bake at 325 degrees Fahrenheit for 15 minutes.

Two Bean Salad

6 servings

1½ can French-cut green beans, drained and rinsed

1½ can yellow wax beans, drained and rinsed

1/4 c. minced green pepper

¼ c. minced red pepper

½ c. minced onion

½ c. salad oil

½ c. cider vinegar

½ c. Stevia

1 tsp. salt

½ tsp. pepper

Place beans in a large bowl. Add green pepper and onion. In a separate bowl, mix oil, vinegar, stevia, salt and pepper. Pour oil mixture over beans and toss until completely covered. Cover and refrigerate overnight.

Zucchini Chips

4 servings

4 zucchini, sliced very thin

¼ c. olive oil

Dry zucchini slices by patting with paper towels. Line slices on baking sheet. Brush slices with olive oil. Bake at 225 degrees Fahrenheit for 2 hours.

Snacks

Banana Raisin Logs

Serving size: 1 banana equals 1 serving

1 banana

2 tbsp. almond butter

2 tbsp. raisins

Peel banana and cut in half. Cut halves in half. Spread 1 tbsp. of almond butter on each half. Sprinkle 1 tbsp. raisins over butter on each half. Top each with plain halves, for little sandwiches.

Brownies

6 servings

10 oz. enjoy life dark chocolate

3 tbsp. coconut oil

1 c. full-fat coconut milk

1 tsp. pure vanilla extract

3 eggs

3 c. almond flour

1/4 tsp. baking soda

1/4 tsp. sea salt

¼ c. chopped walnuts or macadamia nuts, optional

Pre-heat oven to 350 degrees Fahrenheit. In a medium saucepan, over low heat, melt the dark chocolate. (Can also do this very slowly, 1 minute at a time, in the microwave oven, beforehand.) Add to the melted chocolate, coconut oil, coconut milk and vanilla extract. Stir thoroughly together over low heat. Remove mixture and allow to cool completely. In a large bowl, whisk eggs. Add flour, salt and baking soda to the eggs and mix thoroughly. Pour the melted chocolate mixture into g/flour mixture and mix thoroughly, until all lumps are gone. Fold in nuts, if desired. Grease an 8×8 or 9×9 brownie pan with coconut oil. Pour the batter into the pan. Bake for 25 minutes or until a toothpick comes out clean. Cool completely before cutting.

Chocolate Pudding

4 servings

2 ripe avocados

1/2 c. cocoa powder

1/2 c. agave nectar

1/2 c. coconut milk

1 tsp. pure vanilla extract

1/4 salt

Mix all of the ingredients together with a hand mixer until smooth. Pour into small bowls and refrigerate.

Gingerbread Cookies

12 servings

3 c. almond flour

1 tsp. ground ginger

1 tsp. cinnamon

½ tsp. cloves

½ tsp. kosher salt

½ tsp. baking soda

½ c. honey

2 tbsp. pure maple syrup

2 tbsp. melted coconut oil

1 egg

In a medium, bowl mix first six (dry) ingredients together. In a separate bowl, whisk remaining (wet) ingredients together. Pour the wet ingredients into the dry and stir until dough is firm enough to form a ball. Wrap dough in plastic wrap and refrigerate for 4 hours or overnight. On a flat surface place a large piece of parchment paper, Dust the surface and a rolling pin with flour. Roll out the dough until about ¼" thickness. Dust cookie cutter with flour and cut dough into desired shapes. Place cookies on parchment paper-lined baking sheet. Bake at 350 degrees Fahrenheit for 15 minutes. Let cool completely on baking sheet before removing.

Hawaiian Fruit Nut Mix

8 servings

1 c. dried pineapple chunks

1 c. dried apricots

1 c. dried banana chips

1 c. chopped Macadamia nuts

1 c. chopped pecans

1 c. chopped dried dates

1 c. golden raisins

1 c. shredded coconut

In a large bowl, mix all ingredients together.

No-Sugar Sugar Cookies

6 – 8 servings

2 c. almond flour

1/4 tsp. baking powder

3 tbsp. honey

1/8-1/4 tsp. liquid stevia (optional, for sweeter cookies)

1 tbsp. pure vanilla extract

1/4 tsp. sea salt

Preheat oven to 300 degrees Fahrenheit. Line a baking sheet with parchment paper. In a bowl combine and knead all ingredients until firm cookie dough forms. Roll dough into a ball. On a flat surface, sprinkle a little almond flour and turn dough out onto it. Flour a rolling pin and roll the dough out flat to 1/8-1/4 inch thickness. Dust rolling pin, if dough sticks. Dust a little flour on cookie cutters and cut dough into desired shapes, until all dough is used. Place cookies on baking sheet and bake for 19-21 minutes, until bottoms and edges of cookies just become golden brown. Allow cooling slightly and then remove to a wire rack for complete cooling.

Nut & Fruit Mix

6 servings

3 c. cocktail peanuts

2 tbsp. ground cumin

½ tsp. ground ginger

¼ tsp. red pepper

½ c. each banana chips, shredded coconuts, and raisins

Mix all ingredients well.

Red, White & Blue Fruit Snacks

4 servings

1 c. fresh strawberries cut into halves

2 bananas, peeled and sliced into chunks

½ c. fresh blueberries

4 wooden skewers

On a wooden skewer, place a slice of strawberry, a slice of banana, and 1-2 blueberries. Continue stacking and alternating fruit until skewer is full and all fruit is used.